BACKPACKER

Trailside
First Aid

BACKPACKER

Trailside
First Aid

RECOGNITION, TREATMENT, AND PREVENTION

Molly Absolon

Photographs by Dave Anderson

FALCONGUIDES

GUILFORD, CONNECTICUT
HELENA, MONTANA

AN IMPRINT OF GLOBE PEQUOT PRESS

FALCONGUIDES®

Copyright © 2011 by Morris Book Publishing, LLC

Backpacker is a registered trademark of Cruz Bay Publishing, Inc.

FalconGuides is an imprint of Globe Pequot Press.

Falcon, FalconGuides, and Outfit Your Mind are registered trademarks of Morris
Book Publishing, LLC.

Text design: Sheryl P. Kober
Page layout: Melissa Evarts
Project editor: David Legere

Library of Congress Cataloging-in-Publication Data
Absolon, Molly.
 Backpacker magazine's trailside first aid : recognition, treatment, and
prevention / Molly Absolon.
   p. cm.
 ISBN 978-0-7627-5653-7
1. First aid in illness and injury—Handbooks, manuals, etc. 2. Outdoor medical
emergencies—Handbooks, manuals, etc. I. Title. II. Title: Trailside first aid.
 RC86.8.A32 2011
 616.02'52—dc22
                          2010034384

Printed in China
10 9 8 7 6 5 4 3 2 1

Contents

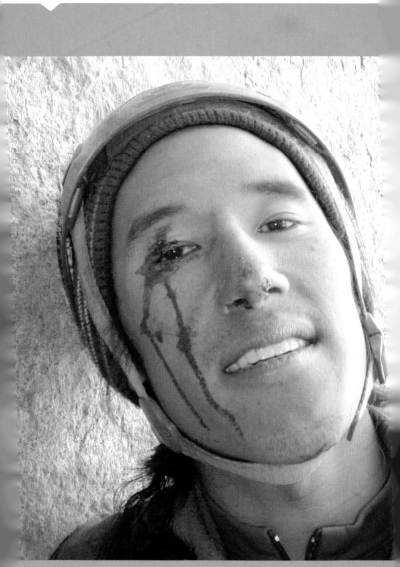

Accidents happen quickly and without warning, so it helps to be prepared.

Introduction

The scream jolted me out of my reverie. Instantly, my heart began to race. I swallowed and paused for a moment before turning around to see what I assumed would be blood and guts, convinced that only something terrible could have caused the sound I'd heard. I reminded myself that I'd been taught to deal with emergencies. I knew what to do: Size up the scene, check for ABCs, stabilize the patient. The list went through my head, soothing me as I ticked off the steps engrained by years of first-aid training.

I turned around. Behind me, one of my backpacking students lay turtled on her back, her arms and legs flailing helplessly in the air as she tried to right herself. Her screams had dissolved into laughter as fear faded into relief and amusement at her ignominious predicament. I relaxed as I realized that we'd escaped. No need for first aid this time. My relief was tempered by a sense of gratitude both for the fact that the student was okay and for the fact that had she not been, I knew what to do.

If you spend a lot of time in the wilderness, you are likely to encounter some kind of first-aid situation. Proper planning helps minimize this likelihood. You can choose routes and activities appropriate for your skill level. You can train to prepare yourself physically. You can carry the appropriate equipment. But you cannot avoid everything. Sometime someone

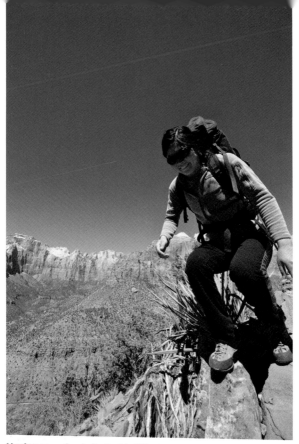

Having some basic first-aid skills allows you to explore the wilderness with confidence.

is going to take a misstep in a boulder field or get a stomachache in camp. You may need to patch a blister or tape an ankle; you may find yourself faced with a broken limb or worse. Having some basic first-aid skills is imperative in these situations, especially when the injured or sick party is someone you love.

HOW TO USE THIS BOOK

By definition, the wilderness is a place far from civilization. You can't pick up the phone, call 911, and expect an ambulance to show up in ten minutes. If someone in your party gets sick or injured, you may have to provide care for hours, if not days, until help

Wilderness first aid includes the ability to care for a patient for hours or days until help arrives.

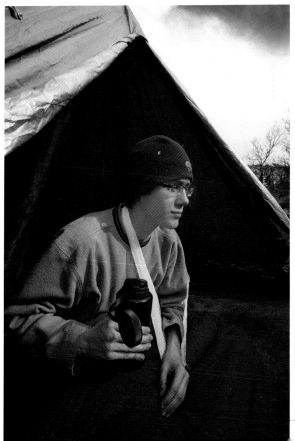

arrives. This book includes basic information for assessing your patient's condition, treating immediate threats to life or limb, caring for minor injuries, and gathering important information to pass on when help arrives.

This book does not provide details on more advanced care or treatments. If you anticipate spending a lot of time in remote wilderness settings, nothing beats having first-aid training. You may never need to use it, but for that moment when you are confronted with a life-or-death situation, having the skills to respond appropriately is worth the time spent in class.

Chapter One

Patient Assessment

The first step in any first-aid situation is to figure out what you are dealing with. Being thorough and methodical in this process is imperative, so first-aid providers have established the following step-by-step guidelines to ensure they don't leave out important information or miss critical clues to their patient's condition.

STEP ONE: SURVEY THE SCENE

Stop, look, and listen before you approach your patient. Your safety is paramount. It may sound ruthless, but if approaching an injured or ill person

Before you approach an injured person, make sure the area is safe.

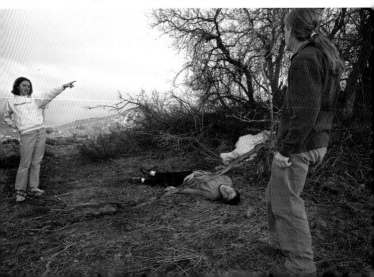

threatens your well-being, you should not proceed. The scene may be too risky: avalanche hazard is high, a fire is out of control, water levels are rising. Throwing yourself blindly into such a situation will only compound the problem.

Sizing up the scene also gives you a chance to look for clues: Your unconscious patient is lying at the base of a tree with a broken branch in her hand, or there's an empty whiskey bottle sitting by his side.

Finally, take a moment to prepare yourself for examining the patient. Body fluids may carry diseases such as HIV or hepatitis. It's best to be cautious and avoid contact. Wear gloves, and consider putting on sunglasses to protect your eyes.

Gloves protect you from blood-borne diseases, so it's a good idea to keep a pair handy in case of an emergency.

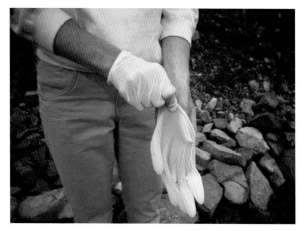

The scene survey should take just seconds: enough time to stop, look around, pull out your first-aid kit, and decide it is safe to proceed.

STEP TWO: INITIAL EXAM—ABCDEs

The initial patient exam is intended to identify immediate threats to life or limb. If you discover something during this exam, you must stop and fix it. The human brain suffers irreversible damage if deprived of oxygen for more than four minutes; likewise, massive arterial bleeding can lead to death quickly if unchecked. You have to act fast to take care of these problems.

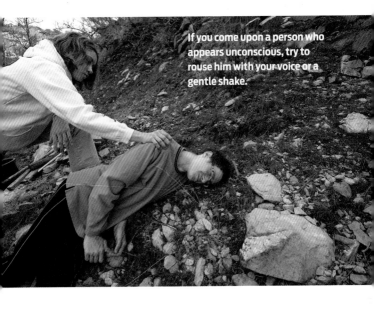

If you come upon a person who appears unconscious, try to rouse him with your voice or a gentle shake.

As you begin performing your assessment, talk to your patient. Introduce yourself if he or she is a stranger. Let the individual know that you are trained and would like to help. Get an okay from her before you begin any kind of treatment. Do this even if your patient appears to be unconscious. Try to wake her by shaking her shoulder and yelling, "Are you okay?" You may find the person has just fallen asleep and is roused by your voice and touch.

ABCDEs

Airway: If your patient is talking, you have an airway, breathing, and a pulse, so you can move on to look for bleeding. If he or she is unconscious, look, listen, and feel for breath sounds. Be patient. Healthy adults breathe between twelve and twenty times per

Get close and give yourself time to look, listen, and feel for breath sounds.

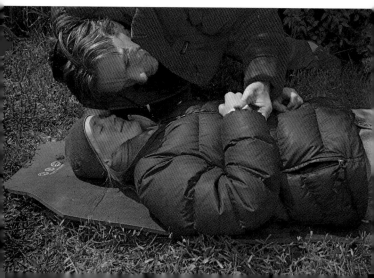

minute, but your breath rate slows when sleeping or cold. Tilt your head close to the patient's mouth and nose; feel for the air against your cheek, watch for the chest to rise and fall. Give yourself ten seconds. If you cannot detect any sign of breathing, open the patient's mouth and look for obstructions: a piece of meat or a candy caught in his throat, or perhaps her tongue has slipped back and blocked her airway.

To open an airway, roll your patient onto her back. Place one hand on her forehead and the other under the bony part of her chin. Tilt her head back and lift her chin.

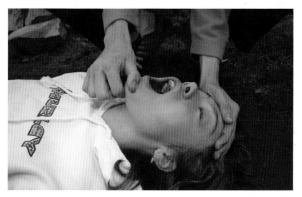

If your patient is not breathing, open her airway using the head-tilt, chin-lift technique. Place one hand on your patient's forehead, the other beneath her chin, and tilt her head back.

If you suspect the patient has injured her spinal cord—something possible with any fall from body height or above—do not move her. Use a jaw thrust

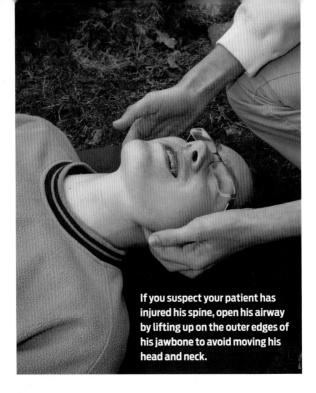

If you suspect your patient has injured his spine, open his airway by lifting up on the outer edges of his jawbone to avoid moving his head and neck.

to open her airway. A jaw thrust is done by placing your fingers under the corners of the individual's jaw and lifting it up and away from her throat.

After opening the airway, look, listen, and feel for breath sounds again. If you do not detect anything, reposition your patient's head and try once more.

Breathing: If you still cannot find any signs of breathing, place your mouth over your patient's, pinch his nose shut, and blow two deep breaths into his lungs. Most first-aid kits include some kind of shield or mask for rescue breathing. If you have one, use it.

Carry a compact face shield in your first-aid kit to protect yourself from germs and bodily fluids if you have to rescue breathe for a patient.

If your patient is not breathing, pinch his nose closed, and breath into his mouth once every five seconds.

Circulation: Once you've checked for breathing, slide your finger down to your patient's throat and feel for a pulse along the side of her jugular. Again, give yourself ten seconds. Heartbeats may be faint, slow, or hard to feel. Don't rush.

If you detect a pulse, great. That means your patient's heart is working. If necessary, continue with rescue breathing, breathing once every five to six

You can find a pulse alongside your patient's jugular.

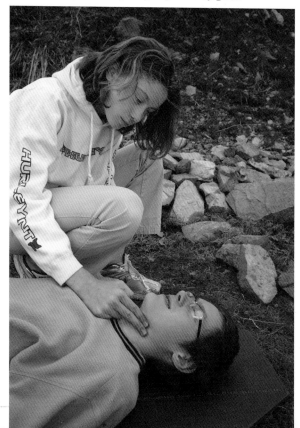

seconds until your patient begins to breathe on her own or help arrives. If you do not detect a pulse and are trained in the technique, consider beginning cardiopulmonary resuscitation (CPR) now.

There are situations in the wilderness where CPR is not recommended. These situations include the following:

» Obvious signs of death or of a lethal injury
» Scene safety concerns
» Frozen patient
» Signs of life such as breathing

You may also be faced with the decision to stop CPR, particularly in the wilderness where medical treatment may be hours away. Justifiable reasons for stopping include exhaustion, lack of response (after thirty minutes or more), or the arrival of a more qualified person who takes over care or pronounces the patient dead.

In addition to checking for pulse, circulation includes looking for bleeding. A patient lying on soft ground or wearing many layers of clothing may not show obvious signs of bleeding. The ground can absorb the blood, or it may be pooled inside a waterproof jacket. Slide your hand under the patient, inside clothing, touch his skin. Open up jackets, look for wounds.

Most bleeding can be controlled by direct pressure and elevation. Take a wad of cloth (ideally sterile

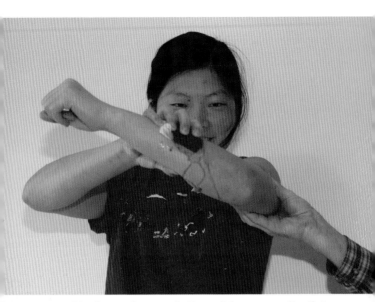

Most bleeding can be controlled by applying pressure directly to the wound, elevating the affected limb, and pressing down on the closest pressure point, in this case the brachial artery in the patient's upper arm.

gauze pads, but anything will do in an emergency) and place it directly over the wound. Press down firmly with the flats of your fingers. Raise the affected body part above the heart. (See Chapter Four for more detail on controlling bleeding.) You can also push on specific pressure points—the brachial artery in the upper arm or the femoral artery in the leg—to slow blood flow into the limb.

Disability: With any patient who appears to have been in some kind of traumatic accident, you should assume a head or spine injury. Moving someone with a spinal cord injury can cause irreversible damage. If you suspect there is a mechanism for such an injury, keep the patient still. Place your hand on his forehead and ask him not to move his head. If the person is lying down, have someone hold his head in place to prevent movement. Or position backpacks, food bags, even padded rocks on either side of the patient's head to keep it still.

Have one person sit and hold your patient's head to keep her still while you examine her.

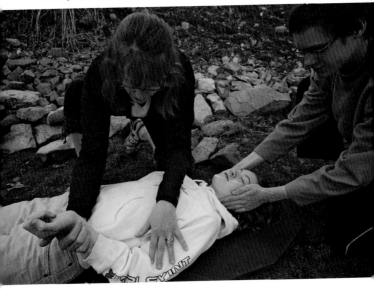

Environment: Finally, you may need to change your patient's environment to protect her from further injury. This includes getting her on an insulated pad, into a sleeping bag, or out of the elements. You may need to erect a tent or create some kind of sunshade—anything to avoid compounding your patient's problem through continued exposure to extreme conditions.

Remember: The initial exam is designed to identify threats to life. If you find a problem during this stage of your assessment, *stop* and *treat* it. Your rapid response can save someone's life.

STEP THREE: THOROUGH PATIENT ASSESSMENT

This part of your patient assessment can be broken down into three parts:

1. Medical history
2. Head-to-toe physical examination
3. Vital signs

It is helpful to have someone take notes. Write down the time, particularly as you record vital signs. You should include negatives. For example, when dealing with a mysterious stomach ailment, it is helpful for the doctor to know not only that the patient is complaining of an aching belly but also that he denies any increased pain when you palpate or press on his abdomen.

1. Medical History

A detailed medical history requires a conscious patient. However, you can get some information from unconscious patients to fill in a few of the blanks. Look in her backpack for medicines. Check wrists, neck, and ankles for medical alert tags. Ask the patient's colleagues if they know anything about her medical condition. When someone is out cold and you have no idea why, any little piece of information can be helpful.

For a conscious patient, your history should proceed as follows:

a. Chief Complaint: What is your patient's primary problem?

A common mnemonic used by first-aid providers for describing a patient's chief complaint is OPQRST:

» **Onset:** Did your patient's problem start suddenly or develop slowly?
» **Provokes:** What caused the injury or how did the illness develop? Do certain activities or positions cause more or less pain?
» **Quality:** How would you describe the type of pain (sharp, dull, throbbing, etc.)?
» **Radiates:** Does the pain move? Can your patient point to a spot and say, "It hurts here"?
» **Severity:** How badly does it hurt? (People often use a 1–10 scale with 10 being the worst

pain the patient has ever felt. Remember, this is a subjective scale. It may help to ask your patient what her worst pain has been in the past.)

» **Time:** When did the pain start? Does it come and go or is it constant? How frequently does it occur if intermittent?

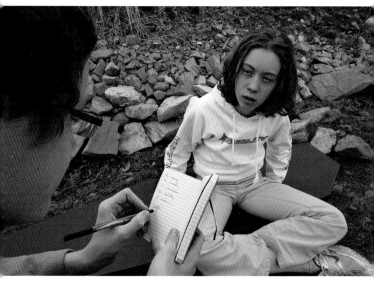

Write down everything. You never know what information might be relevant to your patient's condition.

b. SAMPLE

SAMPLE is a mnemonic used for gathering background information from your patient. It is designed to help you ferret out not only details about her current condition but also things from her past that may be helpful in figuring out what is happening now.

- » **Symptoms:** What are your patient's symptoms? What is she feeling?
- » **Allergies:** Is your patient allergic to anything? If so, is there a chance he was exposed to the allergen? What is his reaction if exposed? This information is also helpful should your patient require medication during treatment.
- » **Medications:** Does the patient use any medications? This should include illegal drugs as well as prescription medications.
- » **Past history:** Does your patient have any medical conditions that you should be aware of? Does he have any relevant history that may add information to the current situation?
- » **Last intake/outtake:** When and what did your patient eat and drink last? How much? Was there anything unusual or noteworthy about his eating and drinking? When was his last bowel movement? Was there anything unusual about that (color, consistency, frequency, smell)? How about the last time he urinated? Again, anything unusual or noteworthy?
- » **Events:** Ask your patient to describe the events that led up to the current situation. Probe a bit here. Look for anything that might be unusual.

2. Physical Exam

With most patients, it's worth conducting a head-to-toe examination to ensure you are aware of any and all potential problems even if it appears that the only issue is a sore leg. Sometimes one injury can mask another. The patient may be so distracted by the pain in one part of her body, she doesn't feel it somewhere else. So take the time to conduct a quick physical exam just in case you are missing something.

Have one person conduct the entire exam for consistency. If you find yourself unsure of whether something feels normal, check the patient's other side or your own body for comparison.

Start at the head and move down to the feet. Palpate using the flats of your fingers. Press gently but firmly. If the patient says, "Ouch," stop pressing, but look at the spot and try to narrow down what caused the pain and how widespread it is. It's important to respect your patient's modesty but critical to inspect them at skin level. Find a private place to conduct your exam. Don't leave them exposed when you are done looking at a spot.

Use all your senses. Smell. Some problems cause unusual breath odors, or a smell may clue you into the presence of alcohol or poison. Look for obvious deformities or discoloration. Watch for guarding or inconsistency. Check for symmetry from one side of the body to the other. Listen for abnormal sounds. Feel for rigidity or swelling.

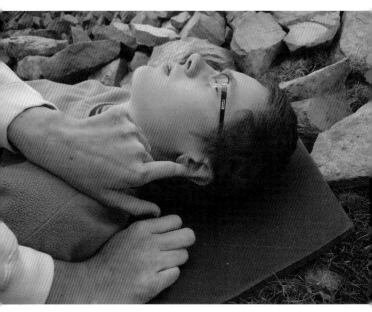

Use all your senses: Look into hidden areas like ears, feel underneath clothing, smell for unusual odors, and listen for unexpected sounds while you conduct your head-to-toe exam.

Make sure you only touch one place at a time so you don't get mixed results. Remember to reach under the patient's body. If you are comfortable having her move (that is, you have no concerns about spinal injuries), have her sit up so you can examine her back.

Divide the abdomen into four quadrants with the belly button marking center and palpate each quadrant individually. This enables you to specify exactly where a patient's pain is located. Remember, when you are talking about right or left, use your patient's right or left, not yours.

Talk to your patient while you conduct your exam. Reassure him and explain what you are doing to help put him at ease.

If you do detect a problem, stop and explore the details with your patient. Can he move the area and what does movement do? Can he wiggle his fingers and toes? Does he detect any tingling sensations?

Write down all the information you gather. You never know what may end up being critical for treatment.

3. Vital Signs

Vital signs are an indicator of our bodies' internal functions: They tell us how our heart, brain, and lungs are doing. These signs can provide clues to what is going on with a patient. They are also invaluable for monitoring someone's conditions over time.

In seriously ill or injured patients, you should monitor vitals every fifteen or twenty minutes. Deteriorating vitals may indicate your patient is going into shock or her condition is worsening.

Level of consciousness: Level of consciousness is measured according to the individual's alertness and her orientation to person, place, time, and events. A conscious patient is by definition awake and alert. Beyond that, we want to determine how alert.

Ask your patient to tell you her name, where she is, what time it is, and what happened. This may repeat questions you've asked before, but it's important to isolate them during your vitals exam to determine level of consciousness accurately. Your patient's level of consciousness will be one of the following in order of deteriorating brain function:

1. Patient knows who she is, where she is, what time it is roughly, and what happened.

2. Patient knows who she is, where she is, what time it is, but cannot recall what happened.

3. Patient knows who she is, where she is, but not what time it is or what happened.

4. Patient knows who she is, but doesn't know where she is, what time it is, or what happened.

5. Patient is alert and awake, but doesn't know who she is, where she is, what time it is, or what happened.

If you have an unconscious patient—or someone who is not awake and alert—you can still determine a bit about her level of consciousness by determining responsiveness. Does the patient groan when you call her name? Does he react if you pinch his arm? Deteriorating responsiveness indicates lower levels of brain function. It may not affect your treatment, but it can tell a doctor a lot.

For non-alert patients, verbal responsiveness indicates the highest level of brain function. Speak loudly to your patient to see if you can elicit any response. Try a couple of times, yell, and watch closely to see if you can pick up a movement: a flicker of an eye, anything to indicate he may have heard your call.

In the absence of a verbal response, try to stimulate the person's brain through pain. Pinch her arm; rub your knuckles into his sternum. Look for a reaction: a groan, a flinch, anything to indicate that pain was felt.

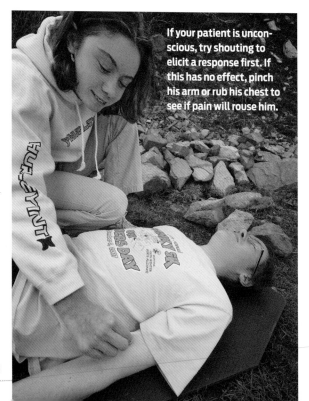

If your patient is unconscious, try shouting to elicit a response first. If this has no effect, pinch his arm or rub his chest to see if pain will rouse him.

Finally, if your patient does not respond to any verbal or pain stimulus, he or she is unresponsive.

Heart rate: Take your patient's pulse. You can find a pulse in a variety of places: The inside of the wrist below the thumb or on the throat next to the jugular are usually the easiest places. The average adult's heart rate is between fifty and ninety beats per minute. Use your watch to get an accurate count. Count for fifteen seconds and then multiply the number by four to determine rate. Describe the quality and rhythm of the beats. A healthy heartbeat is strong and regular; any variations to this should be noted, and includes qualities such as weak, rapid, booming, or irregular.

Respiration rate: Most healthy adults breathe between twelve and twenty times per minute. Check for fifteen seconds and multiply by four to get the total per minute. Be careful. If you tell your patient you are going to count his respirations, there's a good chance he will begin to hold his breath or breathe at an unnatural rate. Your best bet is to take your patient's pulse for fifteen seconds and then, without removing your hand from her wrist, count her respirations for another fifteen seconds.

As with heart rate, the rhythm and quality of respirations is important. Are they labored? Shallow? Rapid? Can you hear any unusual noises? A healthy person's breathing is regular and easy; any changes to that character and rhythm should be recorded.

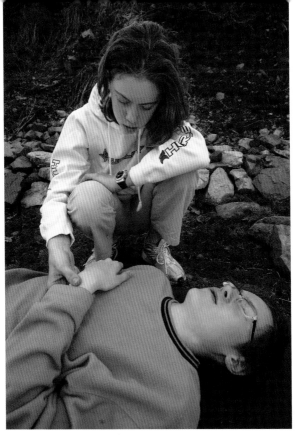

It can be tricky to count respiration rates if your patient is aware of your intention. The best method is to take his pulse with his hand resting on his chest and then count respirations in the same position.

Skin color and temperature: Skin color should be pink. For dark-skinned people, check nail beds or palms for skin color. These areas will be pink in healthy individuals. Changes to skin color indicate changes to blood flow, so, for example, blue or pale skin may mean that blood is not reaching the area. Healthy skin is warm and dry, so note if someone feels hot and sweaty or cold and clammy.

Pupils: Normal pupils are of equal size and respond rapidly to changes in light. To check your patient's pupils, cover her eyes for fifteen to twenty seconds and then remove your hand (in the dark, shine a light briefly in her eyes) to see if the pupils constrict. Any asymmetry or failure to respond to light should be noted.

Temperature: Body temperature is particularly relevant with infections, illness, and with environmental injuries such as heat stroke or hypothermia. You need a thermometer to get an accurate read on body temperature, however, so unless you carry one in your first-aid kit, you may be forced to rely on other signs—levels of consciousness, skin color and temperature, and environmental conditions for example—to indicate elevated or depressed temperatures.

STEP FOUR: WHAT NOW?

Now you should have the situation under control, or at least you've diffused the emergency and bought yourself some time. This time is the big difference between frontcountry first aid and wilderness first aid. Most urban first responders take care of their patient for ten minutes max until the ambulance arrives with paramedics, advanced life support, oxygen, and a direct phone line to the hospital. In the wilderness, you may not see a doctor for a long time.

You now have to make a judgment call. Is this a life-threatening situation? Is your patient about to die? Hard as this may be to accept, if someone is about to die from an injury or illness that demands advanced medical care in the next hour, it is unlikely you can do much more than try to make him comfortable. You may be carrying some kind of communication device—a satellite phone or personal locating beacon—that allows you to call for immediate help. You may even be able to get a helicopter to your side quite rapidly, but it's unlikely it will arrive within an hour unless everything falls into place. You cannot beat yourself up if this is the situation. The wilderness attracts us because it is wild, not safe. You may not be able to do anything to help your patient.

That said, often you can. Now is your time to come up with a plan for what comes next.

SOAP NOTES

SOAP notes are a commonly used format for recording medical information in emergency situations. A SOAP note includes:

- » **S**ubjective information
- » **O**bjective information
- » **A**ssessment
- » A **P**lan

SOAP notes are useful for first-aiders as a guide for organizing their actions and for reporting information to more qualified help.

Subjective information is the stuff your patient tells you: such as his name and his version of events. It includes the patient's age, history of the illness or injury, and the chief complaint (including a description of the associated symptoms).

Objective information is measurable and includes vital signs, results from the head-to-toe exam, and the SAMPLE history.

The **assessment** is your best guess at what is going on. You may not have any medical training, but you've watched enough television over the years to guess that the fifty-year-old man in your party who is describing radiating pain in his chest may be having some kind of heart problem and need immediate medical attention. Likewise, you can guess from the fact that your partner's ankle is the size of a grapefruit and she said she twisted it stepping off a boulder that she has likely sprained or broken the affected joint.

No doctor expects you to be able to diagnose medical problems, but writing down your best guess based on your understanding of the signs and symptoms you've recorded helps the doctor understand where you were coming from. It also helps you determine the urgency of your treatment plan.

There are certain conditions for which you can do very little in the field, such as head, neck, and back injuries; chest injuries; or serious illness. If you suspect any of these problems after conducting your patient exam, you should try to make your patient as comfortable as possible and seek immediate help, whether that means calling out on a satellite phone or radio, running to a road, flagging down another party, or hitting your emergency button on a personal locating beacon.

The **plan** includes everything that happens next. This includes immediate steps—splinting the fractured leg or cleaning the wound—as well as long-term care, such as how you intend to make your patient comfortable until the injury heals or you can get him to a hospital. Can your patient stay with you in the wilderness or does he have to see a doctor? If your patient needs medical attention, can she walk out of the wilderness or are you going to need assistance? What kind of assistance is available? These kinds of questions all need to be addressed in your plan.

The remainder of this book will be dedicated to conditions you can do something about in the field with little medical training.

Chapter Two

Shock

Shock is insidious. Your patient can appear fine, and suddenly she faints and her vital signs plummet. Shock is caused by circulatory system failure. For a number of different reasons ranging from blood loss to severe dehydration or a heart problem, your circulation system fails to deliver adequate oxygen to your body. Untreated, shock causes death.

Shock is associated with other injuries and can be managed—or at least slowed—if recognized. Any time you have someone who has experienced trauma, either physically or emotionally, you should treat for shock.

SIGNS AND SYMPTOMS OF SHOCK

- » Pale, clammy skin
- » Rapid, weak pulse
- » Shallow, rapid respirations
- » Changes in levels of consciousness
- » Thirst
- » Anxiety

TREATMENT

The most important treatment for shock is to remove the cause. This means stopping bleeding, addressing ABCDEs, stabilizing fractures, and alleviating pain as much as possible. Help keep your patient calm by maintaining your personal composure and talking in a soothing, professional manner. If your patient is conscious and capable of holding and drinking from a cup, give him fluids.

Have your patient lie down and prop up his feet with a pillow or some kind of footrest (make sure to support the knees). Ideally, the feet should be approximately 10 inches above the heart. Make sure the patient is comfortable—neither too hot nor too cold. Monitor vitals.

In any traumatic event, you should treat for shock just in case. Have your patient lie down and elevate his feet. Make sure he is comfortable and speak to him in a calm, reassuring voice.

Chapter Three

Fractures, Sprains, and Tendonitis

Athletic injuries, or injuries to the skeletal system and its connective tissues, are one of the most common injuries encountered in the backcountry. People are pushing their physical limits, they may not be in the best shape, they are carrying heavy loads, and the terrain is varied, inconsistent, and unstable. It's easy to fall or step wrong and end up with some kind of injury.

Whether your patient can remain in the wilderness after suffering an athletic injury depends on its severity, but you can definitely do a lot to help her be more comfortable while you come up with a plan.

BONE FRACTURES

Fractures can be open or closed, which means either the skin is broken (open) or intact (closed). Open fractures are very serious. Exposed bones can dry out and the tissue die, plus the opening allows the introduction of bacteria, which can lead to infection. Open fractures demand immediate attention. Clean the wound carefully (see Chapter Four for basic wound care) and keep bone ends moist with a damp dressing. Splint the wound (see sidebar on pages 32–33) and evacuate your patient as soon as possible.

For closed fractures, the threat is less immediate or dire (with the exception of femur fractures; see sidebar on page 36).

Signs and Symptoms

» Mechanism of injury: What happened? Probably the most common sign of a fracture is the simple fact that you fell and heard something snap.
» Deformity: Fractures often result in some deformity. The bones don't line up as they should, or there's a bend where there should not be.
» Discoloration: You may have swelling and discoloration associated with a fracture, but this won't happen immediately, so don't sigh with relief if you don't see it right away.
» Pain and tenderness: Often with fractures, a patient can point out exactly where it hurts.
» Crepitus: You may detect the sound of bones grinding against each other when the injury moves.

Treatment

Once you've identified a fracture, your treatment involves a number of steps. First remove all clothing surrounding the injury. You may need to cut off a sleeve of a shirt or part of a pants leg. You need to see what you are working with, and clothing gets in the way. Remove all jewelry, watches, shoes, and so forth. You are likely to have swelling associated with a fracture, so it's a good idea to get rid of any potentially restrictive items before you no longer can.

Once you have exposed the injury, look to see if the bones are aligned. Most medical professionals now believe you should apply gentle, in-line traction to realign bones if medical attention is distant. To do this, have a helper hold the injured limb above the site of the fracture (this can be the patient if you have no one else to help), while you take hold of the limb below the injury and pull gently until the bone is straight. Stop if the movement is causing more pain.

For a lower arm fracture, apply in-line traction by stabilizing the upper arm with one hand and pulling the lower arm gently until it is straight.

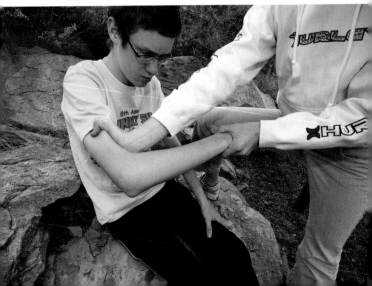

Splinting Made Easy

Splints need to be firm, comfortable, simple, adjustable, and allow access to fingers or toes to check circulation. Most of us don't carry splinting materials in our first-aid kits; there's no need really as the likelihood of encountering a fracture is slim and you can improvise with materials at hand. Everything from spoons to jackets and bandannas, even backpacking seats, can be transformed into an effective splint with a little improvisation.

Firm: You can use a variety of things to provide support to your splint, including rolled foam pads, sticks, tent poles, and so forth. The idea is to have something that prevents movement without being too cumbersome.

Comfortable: Use abundant padding throughout your splint to make sure it is comfortable. Talk to your patient as you work; he will tell you if the splint feels good. If you are unsure, you can experiment on someone else before actually subjecting your patient to the splint. Padding also provides insulation.

Adjustable: Tie your splint in place with wide straps—bandannas, cravats, or strips of cloth from a shirt work well. Use loose knots or even bows that you can untie easily in case the splint needs to be loosened as the limb swells.

Simple: People have a tendency to get a bit carried away with splints. They are fun to build, demanding ingenuity to accomplish their purpose, but they don't have to be too elaborate. The simpler the splint, the easier it is to assess the injury. Splints should be usable. For example, you don't want to splint someone's arm straight out from his side: He could not move in that position without banging into something.

Finally, make sure you leave a window to peep in through so you can check your patient's fingers or toes. You want to make sure he has good skin color and temperature and there is no tingling from lack of blood flow.

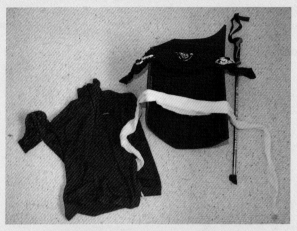

You can improvise a splint from almost anything. Here a shirt, sleeping pad, strip of cloth, and a trekking pole provide materials.

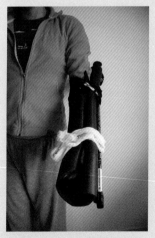

A good splint must be rigid, provide stability, and be comfortable.

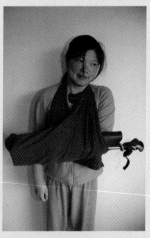

Once you've created your splint, secure the injured arm to your patient with a sling.

Assess the limb for any tingling or numbness to ensure adequate circulation. Make sure to continue checking as you treat.

Immobilize the injury. If you've broken a long bone, you need to also immobilize the joints on either side of the fracture, such as your elbow and wrist if you have a forearm fracture. In the case of a suspected fracture in a joint, immobilize the long bones on either side, such as the upper and lower arm in the case of an elbow injury.

Treat for shock by lying your patient down, comforting him or her, and administering fluids. Fractures may be associated with internal bleeding and extreme pain that can cause shock.

Finally, elevate the limb to help reduce swelling. You can RICE the area (rest, ice, compression, elevation) as well.

Dislocations

Dislocations involve bones being pulled out of the joint sockets. Signs and symptoms of a dislocation include obvious deformity, popping sound at time of accident, extreme pain, and loss of function.

If you take a wilderness first-aid course, you will probably be taught to reduce or fix some dislocated joints in the field—typically patellas, fingers, and shoulders—as it is best to minimize the time a joint is out of alignment both for the patient's comfort and for the long-term health of the joint. If you do not have this training, splint the injury as you find it and get your patient out of the wilderness as quickly as you can.

Evacuation

You'll want to get someone to see a doctor after they have broken a bone, but if you are able to create an effective splint and see no signs of circulation impairment, you can have your patient walk out if they feel up for it (usually this is only possible with

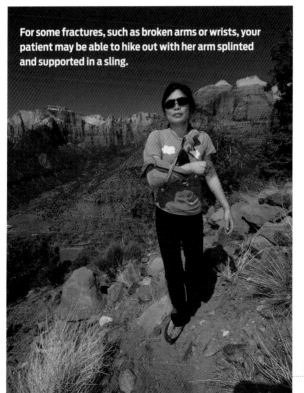

For some fractures, such as broken arms or wrists, your patient may be able to hike out with her arm splinted and supported in a sling.

Femurs

Femur fractures are very serious because of the size of the muscles in your thigh, which can contract, drawing bone ends together and causing pain. Femur fractures can also cause extensive internal bleeding. The recommended treatment for a femur fracture is a traction splint, which requires training to construct. In the absence of this training, you can hold manual traction on a femur fracture by grabbing the patient's foot and pulling hard in line with the long bones. The critical thing is once traction is applied, you do not want to stop, but holding a femur in-line is exhausting. You can tie something around your patient's ankle and foot and secure it to a tree to hold traction until help arrives. Treat all femur fracture patients for shock.

You can provide traction for a femur fracture by tying the patient's injured leg to a tree.

arm or shoulder injuries, but some people can hobble out with makeshift crutches or leaning on others for lower leg fractures).

If you are unable to maintain adequate circulation or if the patient shows signs and symptoms of shock, you need to expedite your evacuation process to ensure your patient's continued well-being.

SPRAINS

Sprains involve injuries to your connective tissues: your tendons and ligaments. Severe sprains are impossible to distinguish from fractures without an X-ray, so in the field if you can't tell, immobilize the area.

Sprains are graded according to severity and range from minor ligament stretches to complete tears. A severe sprain can take months to heal, but a minor sprain may be usable after RICE.

Assessing a Sprain

In the wilderness the most common sprains you can expect to encounter will be ankle sprains. Again, your first clue will be the mechanism of injury. Did the person roll her ankle on the trail? Did he hear a popping sound and feel a flash of pain? Those signs pretty clearly indicate a sprain or possibly a fracture, while pain that comes on slowly is likely to be caused by overuse (see tendonitis on page 41).

Sprains are also associated with discoloration, swelling, and pain. Deformity and point tenderness, on the other hand, point to a fracture. If you suspect a sprain, ask your patient to move the joint; point and flex her toes and rotate her foot in a circle in both directions. You may find that she has lost some range of motion and that certain movements cause pain while others do not. If the person can bear weight and endure a certain amount of use, you may be able to treat the injury in the field.

Treatment

Begin RICE (rest, ice, compression, and elevation) immediately. Apply ice or snow wrapped in a towel or T-shirt to the injury for twenty to forty minutes every two to four hours for the first day or two to help reduce swelling. You can also stick the injured limb in a cold mountain stream to achieve the same result. Your goal is to constrict blood flow and numb nerve pain to help minimize inflammation.

» Wrap the limb in an elastic bandage to apply compression. Make sure the bandage does not cut off blood flow to the limb.

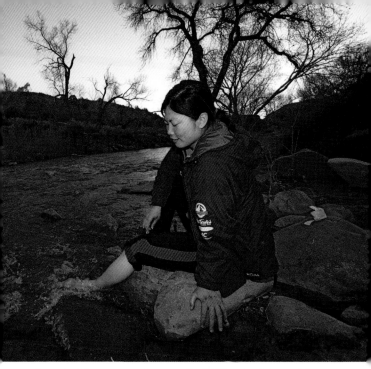

If you don't have snow or ice to use for RICEing your injury, stick the affected area into a cold stream for the same effect.

» Elevate the affected area above the heart to reduce blood flow and help lessen swelling.
» Administer an over-the-counter analgesic such as ibuprofen or acetaminophen to help control pain, and have the patient move the joint (circles, flexing, pointing) gently every few hours. Avoid movements that cause excessive pain.

Taping Ankles

For minor to moderate ankle sprains, you can use tape to stabilize and support the joint enough to allow your patient to continue hiking if he or she desires.

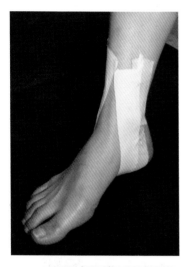

Most ankle sprains occur when you roll your ankle to the outside. You can support this injury by taping the ankle. Start by creating stirrups that begin on the inside of your ankle, pass under your heel, and come up on the out—or injured—side.

To provide further support, create two or three "figure eights" over the stirrups using a strip of tape. Start at the back of the ankle, cross over the top of the foot, pass under the arch, and back over the top of the foot, ending in the back of the ankle where you started.

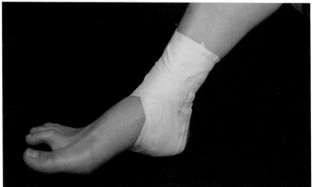

TENDONITIS

Tendonitis, or the inflammation of a tendon, is relatively common on extended hiking or kayaking trips because of the repetitive nature of the activity. Tendonitis is usually—though not always—an overuse injury and in walkers is experienced in the knees and Achilles tendons. Boaters commonly get tendonitis in their wrists.

Signs and Symptoms

Tendonitis may cause some swelling, but often the main signs will be tenderness, pain with movement, and in few cases, a kind of crackly or grinding feeling in the area. Typically, tendonitis comes on slowly.

Treatment

Start with RICE and analgesics to control pain. You can also experiment with different techniques to limit motion in the joint or remove pressure on the tendon. Heel lifts can help with Achilles tendonitis as can changing your shoes to remove any pressure on the tendon. Taping wrists for forearm tendonitis can help reduce the movement that causes pain for boaters. You may be forced to abstain from the activity that causes the pain until the inflammation goes down.

It's worth noting that tendonitis is often associated with technique. You may be someone who rocks back and forth on your feet when you walk, causing a lot of motion in your ankle joint, or you may flex your wrists too much when boating, putting undue pressure on the tendons in your forearm. Try walking flat-footed or switching to a non-feathered paddle to help avoid the motion that is causing pain.

A FEW FINAL THOUGHTS ON ATHLETIC INJURIES

Athletic injuries happen more commonly when people are cold, tired, dehydrated, and out of shape. You can help avoid this situation by warming up for activities, maintaining adequate hydration, resting, and making sure you are prepared.

Chapter Four

Wound Management

Cuts, scrapes, and blisters are common in the outdoors and usually don't cause problems if they are cared for properly. But failure to keep these wounds clean can result in infection, and suddenly an insignificant bug bite turns into a medical emergency, so it's important to treat every opening in your skin seriously.

Small cuts and scrapes—common in the outdoors—can become dangerous if not treated with care to avoid infection.

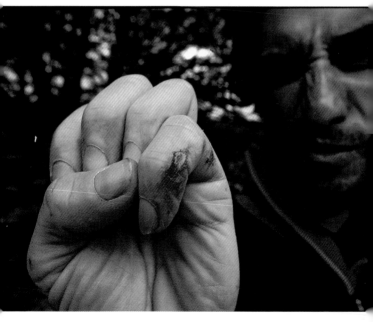

BLEEDING

As mentioned in Chapter One, most bleeding can be controlled by:

» Direct pressure
» Elevation
» Pressure points

Remember to wear gloves or place your hand in a plastic bag when you are around someone else's blood. You may need to apply direct pressure for a long time before the bleeding stops. Check the wound after a minimum of five minutes to see if clotting has occurred; if not, hold the dressing in place for another ten or fifteen minutes and then check again. Back up your direct pressure with elevation and pressure points: Together, you should be able to control most bleeding.

There are situations—usually tears of major arteries—where bleeding cannot be controlled by these techniques. In such extreme situations, you are advised to use a tourniquet. Tourniquets cut off all blood to the limb, so you risk permanent damage if they remain in place for extended periods of time.

Tourniquets should be placed 2 inches above the wound. Wrap a wide band around the limb, tie an overhand knot, place a stick on the knot, and tie it in place with another overhand knot. Twist the stick until bleeding stops and secure. Write TK on

Pressure points are areas where major arteries run close to bones, such as in the upper arm or in the groin area. You can reduce blood flow to the limb below the point by pushing the artery up against the bone, thereby restricting the amount of blood moving through. Once the wound has stopped bleeding, gradually reduce the pressure on the artery allowing blood flow to return to normal slowly. If bleeding resumes, start the process over again.

For major wounds, it can take anywhere from 5 to 20 minutes to stop the blood flow, so be patient.

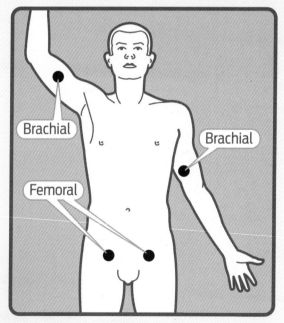

Pressure points of the body

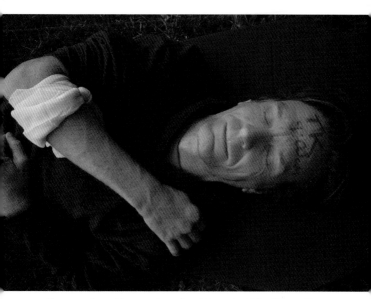

If you are forced to use a tourniquet to control bleeding, write the time and TK on your patient's forehead so the attending physician will know immediately to look for the tourniquet.

your patient's forehead so treating physicians know immediately to look for the tourniquet. Seek immediate evacuation.

For serious wounds, leave the injury alone after you have controlled the bleeding and seek medical attention as quickly as possible. Trying to clean these injuries will just restart the bleeding. For less serious wounds, or wounds where bleeding is minor, your next step is to clean the area.

CLEANING WOUNDS

Infection is a serious problem in the wilderness, so it's imperative that you keep all wounds clean. For most wounds, the best cleaning technique is to flush the area with water that is safe to drink. It's a good idea to carry a syringe in your first-aid kit to irrigate wounds with sufficient pressure, but if you don't have one, a clean plastic bag with a tiny hole in one corner will suffice. Hold the edges of the wound

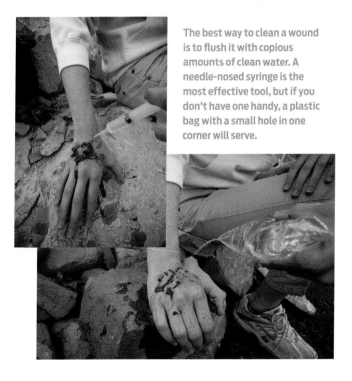

The best way to clean a wound is to flush it with copious amounts of clean water. A needle-nosed syringe is the most effective tool, but if you don't have one handy, a plastic bag with a small hole in one corner will serve.

apart, and tilt the limb slightly so water can flow out. Flush the wound with a continuous high-pressure flow. Use about 0.5 liter and then stop and examine the injury. Pick out any bits of dirt, gravel, or sticks with sterilized tweezers. Flush the area again with another 0.5 liter.

You usually don't have to use any kind of disinfectant or soap if you use an adequate amount of water. Many disinfectants, such as povidone-iodine, are actually fairly caustic even when diluted. If you have a particularly dirty wound or are worried about germs, say from an animal bite, you may want to clean with disinfectant. Just make sure to flush out the wound thoroughly with clean water afterward to remove all trace of the disinfectant.

Some wounds, such as abrasions, need scrubbing to get really clean. You can use a soap-impregnated sponge, available from first-aid suppliers, or a sterile gauze pad and soap for scrubbing. It may help to give your patient some mild analgesic twenty minutes or so before the cleaning to help dull the pain. It may also help to have him do the scrubbing himself if he's up for it. Pick out large foreign objects with tweezers first, scrub, and then irrigate thoroughly.

Once the wound is clean, let it air-dry. If you have a gaping injury and are carrying steri-strips in your first-aid kit, use the strips to pull the wound together or improvise with strips of athletic tape. Start in the middle and work out toward the ends, interlacing strips from one side of the wound to the other like a zipper to help pull it together evenly.

Well-stocked first-aid kits often include occlusive dressings such as Tegaderm that help keep the wound moist, promoting healing. If you don't have such dressings, apply antibacterial cream to a sterile pad and place it over the cut. Use athletic tape to hold the dressing in place.

Check the fingers or toes on the affected limb to make sure you have not cut off circulation. If bleeding resumes, do not remove the dressing as you'll destroy any clotting. Add more dressing material to soak up further blood.

If you use an occlusive dressing on the wound, you can leave it in place for several days. Many of these dressings are see-through, allowing you to

An occlusive dressing keeps your wound clean and dry, and allows you to monitor the area for infection.

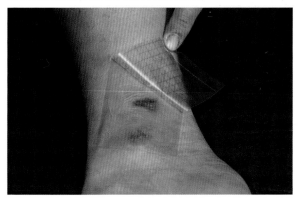

monitor for infection without disrupting healing. They are also waterproof, helping to maintain an ideal healing environment. In the absence of an occlusive dressing, try to keep the bandage and dressing dry. Change the bandage every day or so to help prevent infection. If the dressing is stuck to the wound, soak the area until you can remove it without ripping off scabs.

Infection

Signs of infection include increased redness, heat, swelling, and pain. As the infection becomes more serious, you may see red streaking leading away from the wound toward the heart; lymph nodes swell and your patient may develop a fever. Ideally, you won't get that far, however. Most localized infections can be treated easily if caught early.

Your first step for treating an infection is to reclean the wound. You'll need to open it up or remove scabs to clean effectively. Soak the wound in warm water or antiseptic solution for twenty to thirty minutes several times during the day. Rinse with water that is safe to drink after each soak. Air-dry and redress.

Watch for signs of the infection worsening. Some people carry antibiotics specifically for skin infections, particularly when they travel overseas or expect to be far from medical care for an extended period of time. If you are carrying antibiotics for this purpose, administer them if you begin to see signs of deepening infection. Fever, red streaks, and swollen lymph nodes are all reasons to get your patient to a doctor as soon as possible. Infections on the face are particularly risky and merit rapid medical attention if they do not improve with cleaning.

BURNS

Burns are problematic in the field for a number of reasons: They are prone to infection, they can be extremely painful, and they can cause swelling, which may threaten airways if in the throat area.

Treating Burns

The first step in treating all burns is to remove the source. If your patient is on fire, have him stop, drop, and roll. Burns from wet caustic chemicals should be flushed with water for twenty minutes; dry chemicals should be brushed off the skin.

Once the source of the heat is removed, cool the burned area by pouring water over the burn. You can also use a cool, damp cloth for this purpose. Cool the area for several minutes.

Next, assess the injury. Burns are graded according to their depth and extent, with superficial burns involving only the outer skin layers being the least serious. Superficial burns do not involve blistering, but they are painful, as anyone who's had a good sunburn will know. Partial-thickness burns are more serious and cause blistering. These burns appear wet and mottled, and are very painful. Full-thickness burns go all the way through your skin layers into the subcutaneous. Full-thickness burns appear gray and charred. They may be less painful than other burns because the nerves have been destroyed, but often your patient will have partial-thickness burns as well so don't expect him to be pain free.

Superficial burns can be treated in the field, as can small, localized partial-thickness burns. Burns to the hands, feet, face, or genital area and burns that go all the way around a limb, as well as burns covering a large area, are more serious and should be attended to by a doctor. Cover the burned area with a moist dressing (Second Skin works well for this), treat for shock, and seek help.

BLISTERS

Blisters are friction burns and are common injuries for hikers wearing new boots or covering long miles. Unfortunately they can put a serious glitch in your travel plans. Big blisters make walking uncomfortable or even impossible. Your best bet is to nip any blister in the bud. You'll know when something's going on: Most blisters start with a "hot spot" where the rubbing occurs. Stop and fix the problem right away.

Often blisters can be avoided by wearing comfortable, well-broken-in footwear and clean socks.

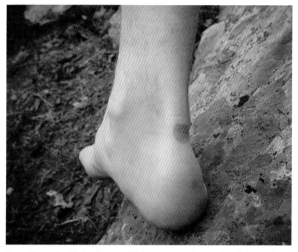

Stop if you feel heat from rubbing on your feet while hiking. A hot spot is easier to treat than an actual blister.

But some people's feet are softer and more prone to blisters, and all shoes and boots are new at some point, so blisters happen. If you catch the injury at the hot spot stage, you're lucky. Today you can buy gel blister pads that pad the area and remove the friction, preventing the actual blister from forming. If you know you are prone to blisters, say on your heel, you may want to put one of these blister gel pads on the sensitive spot prophylactically. They aren't cheap but they work.

You can also use gel pads to cover small liquid-filled blisters, but if the blister is large, you may need to drain the area before you cover it up. The blister will pop once you start walking anyway, so draining it with a sterilized needle is a bit more controlled. After the blister is drained, clean the wound, bandage it, and watch for infection. If you have some kind of foam padding (mole foam or an ensolite pad will work), you can make a doughnut to surround the affected area, remove the friction, and help alleviate pain.

A doughnut made from mole foam can be used to stop the rubbing that caused your blister.

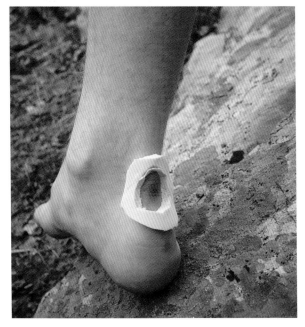

Chapter Five

Stings and Bites

One of the things we all complain about when we go camping is the bugs. Whether it's the mosquitoes in the Rockies or blackflies in Maine, bugs can be simply annoying or they can be a health hazard. Insects can carry diseases or inject venom, so it's worth knowing what is out there. Snakes and mammals can also pose a risk. Specific animal and insect hazards vary around the world; for this book we'll just address the problems you may encounter in North America.

MOSQUITOES

The whining buzz of mosquitoes provides a constant backdrop on many summer backpacking trips. The spread of West Nile virus—a mosquito-borne illness that can make you quite ill—has changed the seriousness with which we take their presence in many parts of the United States. Nowadays, it's worth covering up and using bug repellent to avoid exposure. DEET has been proven effective at keeping mosquitoes at bay, but it has a strong odor that puts many people off as well. You can also use a repellent called picaridine, which is sold under the trade name Bayrepel or Saltidin. Picaridine has been used in Europe and

Australasia for a while and is proven to be as effective as DEET without the odor. Both products are considered safe for human use.

In addition to using repellent, try to avoid exposure during peak times of mosquito activity, especially around dusk. Wear headnets and sleep in netting or under tents in mosquito country. Children can be very sensitive to mosquito bites, so take care to cover them up well. Kids also have a hard time refraining from scratching, so you may want to include some kind of anti-itch cream in your first-aid kit if you anticipate lots of bug bites.

TICKS

Ticks are nasty little critters. They suck your blood and then regurgitate yucky, germ-laden stuff into your body that can make you very sick. Ticks are the leading carriers of disease to humans in the United States, second only to mosquitoes worldwide. They carry Rocky Mountain spotted fever, Lyme disease, and Colorado tick fever.

The best way to avoid ticks is to stay away from them, but that may mean staying inside all summer, which most people don't want to do.

You may not win any style points, but tucking your pants into your socks and wearing light-colored clothing can help minimize your exposure to disease-carrying ticks. ▶

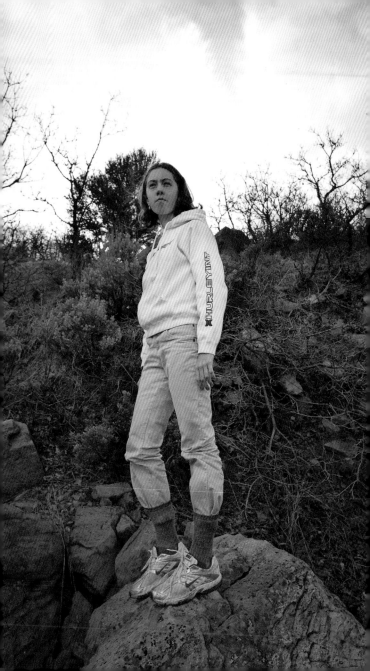

In lieu of total avoidance, you can do the following to limit your exposure:

» Wear light-colored, long-sleeved shirts and pants, and tuck your pants legs into your socks. The light color allows you to detect ticks on your body more easily.
» Use insect repellent (check to make sure the product is effective against ticks).
» Conduct frequent tick checks. Focus attention on warm, dark places: groin, armpits, around ears, and along your hairline.

Tick bites are often painless, so you may not even know you've been bitten. If you do find a tick attached to your body, remove it by pulling back gently and firmly. Once the tick is off, clean the area thoroughly.

Keep tabs on your health over the next few weeks. Even if you don't see a tick on your body, if you develop an unexplained fever, rash, numbness, weakness, or swelling and pain in your joints after spending time in tick country, let your doctor know you may have been bitten.

BEES AND WASPS AND ANAPHYLAXIS

For most of the population, bee stings are simply uncomfortable, but for a significant number of people, they cause an extreme allergic reaction called anaphylaxis, which can be deadly. Anaphylaxis can also be caused by exposure to other allergens: peanuts, shellfish, and certain medications are common culprits.

For the basic bee or wasp sting, the quicker you can remove the stinger, the less intense your reaction will be. Scrape or flick the stinger away and clean the wound. Ice or cold compresses can help alleviate pain, which usually goes away quickly. You may experience continued itching for a day or two.

If you experience a more intense reaction to a sting—or you receive multiple stings at the same time—you may want to administer an antihistamine to help calm your body's reaction. A moderate reaction will cause swelling, itching, and hives.

Anaphylaxis typically occurs within thirty minutes of exposure. Signs of an anaphylactic reaction include hot, burning skin; hives; elevated pulse; anxiety; and most importantly, increasing respiratory distress. Most people who die from anaphylaxis die from respiratory failure. Your treatment needs to be immediate. Calm your patient; give her oral antihistamines and, if necessary, inject epinephrine.

Victims often have a history of allergic reactions, but not always. If you have had a moderate reaction to bee stings in the past, you should carry some kind of bee-sting kit containing injectable epinephrine as a precaution. Epinephrine is a prescription drug. If anyone in your party is prone to allergies, it is worth talking to his or her doctor about securing a prescription just in case. If you know you are going to be traveling in an area with a lot of wasps and bees, you may also want to consider talking to your doctor about carrying epinephrine.

SNAKES

Snakes freak us out, but the reality is bees and wasps kill a lot more people than snakes do. Most bites occur when snakes are provoked. People try to pick them up or they poke at them to get a reaction. Your best way to avoid a bite is to leave snakes alone.

That said, you can't always see snakes. They like to be hidden under ledges or bushes, and their colors are often muted and camouflaged. It can be helpful to walk with a stick in snake country so you can poke under stuff before you step down. Snakes feel vibrations, so walk heavily to alert them to your presence and don't blindly shove your hand into dark, sheltered places.

North America has two types of venomous snakes: Elapidae, or coral snakes, and Crotalidae, or pit vipers, including rattlesnakes, copperheads, and water moccasins. Coral snakebites are rare as the animals are not aggressive and their fangs are short, making it difficult for them to bite humans. Unlike pit viper venom, coral snake venom is a neurotoxin; however, treatment is the same for both kinds of bites with one notable exception. For coral snakebites, place a wide elastic band directly over the bite site.

Otherwise, treatment for snakebites is to follow these steps:

1. Calm your patient.
2. Remove jewelry, watches, and restrictive clothing, and immobilize the affected limb. Do not elevate the injury. Medical opinions vary on whether the area should be lower or level with the heart, but the consensus is that it should not be above it.
3. Make a note of the circumference of the limb at the bite site and at various points above the site as well. This will help you monitor swelling.
4. Evacuate your victim. Ideally he should be carried out to minimize movement. If the victim appears to be doing okay, he can walk. Stop and rest frequently, and if the swelling appears to be spreading or the patient's symptoms increase, change your plan and find a way to get your patient transported.
5. If you are waiting for rescue, make sure to keep your patient comfortable and hydrated (unless he begins vomiting).

Snakebite treatment is rife with old-fashioned remedies: You used to be told to cut and suck the venom out of the bite site or to use a suction cup extractor for the same purpose; applying an electric shock to the area was even in vogue for a while. Do not do any of these things. Do not apply ice, do not give your patient painkillers, and do not apply a tourniquet. All you really want to do is keep your patient calm and get help.

MAMMAL BITES

Mammal attacks are rare, but if you are bitten by an animal, you should seek immediate medical attention. Bites can be very dirty and ragged, hard to clean, and prone to infection. Rabies may be a concern (especially if you are bitten by a skunk or raccoon), so the faster you seek help, the better your prognosis.

The other significant mammal-related concern in North America is hanta virus, which has been associated with inhalation of dried rodent droppings. Hanta virus is a respiratory illness that can be quite severe, even life threatening. To avoid exposure, take care not to crawl around or disturb rodent dens. Avoid camping in areas where rodent droppings are present.

Chapter Six

Heat and Cold Illnesses

We lose heat through four basic mechanisms: conduction, convection, radiation, and evaporation. Conduction occurs when our warm body comes in contact with something cold: Heat naturally travels from the warm body to the cold one. Convection results from heat being moved away from our bodies by water or wind. Radiation is the output of our body's basic metabolic processes: We radiate off the heat that we generate from moving, breathing, living. Finally, evaporation is our way of getting rid of excess heat. We sweat out moisture that evaporates off our skin, cooling us down.

Understanding these mechanisms is important so you can dress appropriately for all conditions.

Avoiding heat or cold injuries also involves behavior modification. It's no coincidence that southern cultures shut down at midday for a siesta. Avoiding the hottest part of the day is smart when the temperature soars above 90°F. Staying comfortable without the help of a furnace or air-conditioning is a constant game. You're always pulling a layer out of your pack or stuffing one back in as you try to maintain a comfortable temperature.

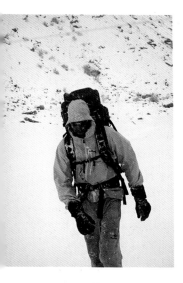

You need to dress for the conditions to ensure you stay warm and dry regardless of the weather.

But sometimes we fail. One of the most common camping injuries is mild hypothermia. Recognizing the signs and symptoms of both cold and heat injuries is important for those times when you—and your partners—wait a bit too long to layer up or cool down.

HYPOTHERMIA

Hypothermia is a continuum of symptoms: As you get colder, the symptoms multiply and worsen. Initially, you'll probably only notice you have trouble zipping your jacket or buttoning a coat. Your fingers don't work quite right. You shiver and feel lethargic. This stage is considered mild hypothermia and is usually easy to reverse.

Have your patient change into dry clothes or seek shelter from the elements. Get him to move around. Do fifty jumping jacks, sprint across a field, run in place. You can give him a hot sugary drink like cocoa followed by a meal. Often hypothermia is associated with fatigue and hunger, commonly occurring at the end of a long, hard day out in the rain and cold. So changing those conditions and helping your patient get warm, fed, and rested is usually all you need to counter mild hypothermia.

As a person cools down further, her symptoms will continue to deteriorate. Moderate hypothermic patients aren't just challenged by zippers and buttons; they also become uncoordinated and have trouble walking. Your patient may not make much sense when she talks; she may be uncooperative, withdrawn, lethargic, or possibly aggressive. These changes in levels of consciousness will continue to deteriorate as the patient cools. You need to stop the process as quickly as possible to prevent having someone slip into severe hypothermia.

Get the individual out of wet clothes and into a sleeping bag. Swaddle the sleeping bag in a windproof, waterproof ground cloth or tent fly to create a vapor barrier for trapping in all heat. Give the patient hot water bottles to place next to his groin and armpits (take care to cover the bottles in a sock or cloth so they don't burn the skin). For most moderately hypothermic patients, this treatment will be enough to rewarm them and bring them out of danger. Beware, however. A recently rewarmed hypothermic patient is fragile and can easily cool down again. He will need rest, food, and fluids before he can resume normal activities.

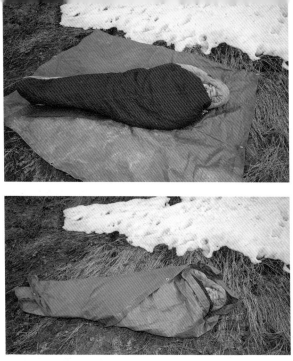

A hypo-wrap made from a sleeping bag wrapped in a windproof tarp can be an effective way to rewarm a moderately hypothermic patient.

Severely hypothermic patients are so cold they become catatonic. They may appear dead. Their heart rate slows and they are unresponsive. These patients are unstable. Their hearts can easily be sent into defibrillation by sudden movements, so extreme care must be taken when transporting them. If you find yourself with a severely hypothermic individual, gently wrap her in a sleeping bag to try to prevent further heat loss and call for immediate help. She needs to be rewarmed in a hospital.

FROSTBITE

When temperatures drop below freezing, frostbite becomes a concern. Frostbite is frozen tissue and, like burns, is categorized by its depth. Superficial frostbite, or frostnip, affects the outermost layers of skin. It usually presents itself as a white spot on the tip of your nose or cheek. You can take care of the problem by holding your hands to your face and blowing to warm the area. But if you return to the conditions that caused the freezing in the first place, you'll get nipped again. Make sure you cover your face when the wind blows and temperatures fall to protect yourself against frostnip.

More serious are partial-thickness and deep frostbite. Partial-thickness frostbite appears white, mottled, or gray. The surface tissue feels hard. Blisters appear after rewarming. Partial-thickness frostbite commonly occurs on fingers and toes—areas that are hard to keep warm in extreme conditions. If your feet or hands go numb, stop and fix the problem before they freeze. Stick the cold area on someone's belly; swing your arms or legs until you feel them begin to warm. Rewarming will be painful when you are really cold, so you'll know right away if your treatment is working. If you are traveling with children or inexperienced adults, you may want to check their hands and feet periodically to make sure they aren't getting too cold.

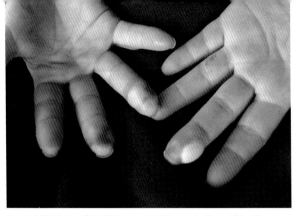

Partial-thickness frostbite causes blisters to form after the area is rewarmed.

If the area actually freezes, you need to rewarm it rapidly by immersing it in warm water (100°F to 108°F) to ensure proper healing.

Deep frostbite, as the name indicates, goes deeper into the tissue and may involve muscle. Frostbite this severe can cause lasting complications, including the loss of fingers and toes. The signs of deep frostbite are similar to those of partial-thickness frostbite: gray, mottled, or white. But the area may feel wooden or frozen. After rewarming, deep frostbite victims will often have large, blood-filled blisters.

As with partial-thickness frostbite, deep frostbite should be rewarmed by immersing the affected area in warm water. Water temperature has to remain above 100°F throughout the process, which is challenging when you have a big chunk of ice in it! You'll need a continuous source of warm water to maintain the heat.

If you've ever experienced the tingling, searing pain of rewarming cold hands, you can imagine the sensation rewarming a frozen limb will cause. This treatment hurts. You may want to give your patient some kind of analgesic—ibuprofen or acetaminophen—to help dull his pain.

Rewarming frostbite is difficult to do properly in the field. You do not want to rewarm a frozen limb and then allow it to freeze again. A cycle of freezing and thawing, freezing and thawing increases tissue damage and can cause permanent problems. Therefore, you may choose to have your patient hike out without rewarming a frostbitten area so that you can rewarm it in the controlled environment of your home or a hospital. Be careful, however; hiking generates heat and can also trigger rewarming. Try to keep the area cold by removing clothing or adjusting your pace.

After the area has rewarmed, the tissue is sensitive. Try to keep blisters intact. Remove any jewelry or constrictive clothing, as the area will swell. Again, ibuprofen or acetaminophen can help manage pain.

IMMERSION FOOT

Prolonged exposure to damp, cool conditions can cause nerve damage in your feet. Immersion foot is a non-freezing injury. Blood flow to the affected area is reduced as a result of vessel constriction, causing oxygen and nutrient deprivation.

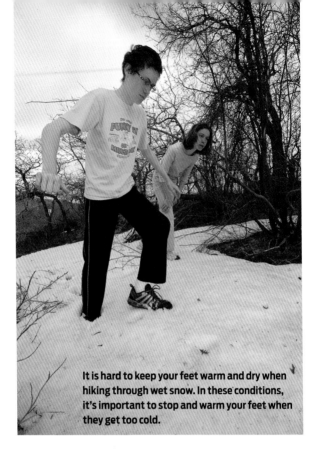

It is hard to keep your feet warm and dry when hiking through wet snow. In these conditions, it's important to stop and warm your feet when they get too cold.

The way to avoid immersion foot is to keep your feet warm and dry. Do not tolerate cold feet. Stop and warm them during the day, especially when hiking in cold, wet conditions, such as through snow. Keep a warm, dry pair of socks in your backpack for sleeping. Dry out socks throughout your trip by wearing them on your shoulders under backpack straps while hiking or sleeping with them at night.

Conventional wisdom is that immersion foot takes awhile to come on, but evidence indicates that as little as three hours of exposure to cold, wet conditions can cause damage. So be aggressive. Model proactive behavior by taking off your boots at rest stops and warming up cold toes. If you need to, stick your feet on someone's belly for some extra help.

Affected feet may appear gray and mottled and feel wooden, but not all people exhibit these signs. Immersion foot often does not show itself until you are out of the mountains and into a hot shower.

Sometimes the best way to warm someone's feet is to put them on a warm belly.

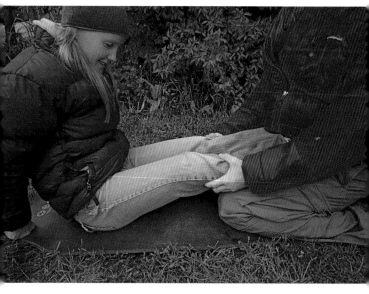

Suddenly your feet are burning and stinging. They may turn bright red and throb. The pain of immersion foot can be incapacitating. You can try taking analgesics, but many immersion foot sufferers say they do not help. Your main treatment is to keep your feet warm and dry and wait it out. Elevate your feet to minimize swelling.

HEAT EXHAUSTION AND HEAT STROKE

At the opposite end of the temperature spectrum are heat injuries. Bodies that become too hot do not do well. When ambient temperatures soar up into the 90s and above and humidity increases, you need to be aware of the potential for heat exhaustion or heat stroke. Modify your activities. Avoid exertion during the hottest parts of the day. Wear cool, light-colored cotton clothing and a sun hat. Seek shade, drink plenty of water, and eat salty snacks.

Heat exhaustion and heat stroke may come on progressively, with an individual gradually deteriorating from one into the other, or they may be entirely separate. Heat stroke occurs when body temperatures soar above 104°F. It can be deadly. Heat stroke victims have a rapid pulse and hot, red skin; they may be delirious or comatose. They are in extreme danger and need to be in a hospital as quickly as possible.

Heat exhaustion is indicated by weakness, nausea or vomiting, headache, fatigue, vertigo, and thirst.

Treatment for both heat stroke and heat exhaustion is to remove the victim from the heat. Get her into the shade and lying down; place cool, damp cloths on her forehead to help cool her. Hydrate. If you have a thermometer, monitor her temperature. Evacuate if you suspect heat stroke.

Overheated patients need to get into the shade, drink fluids, and rest to recover.

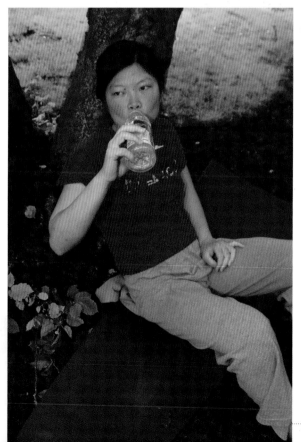

Like hypothermic patients, individuals who have suffered from heat exhaustion will not be able to resume normal activity levels immediately. They are often extremely tired and need time to rest, rehydrate, and eat.

HYPONATREMIA

You can drink too much water, especially if you are exerting yourself in hot temperatures and sweating a lot. In this situation, too much water and not enough salt can cause an electrolyte imbalance known as hyponatremia. Hyponatremia is serious and requires medical help. Your best treatment is to avoid the condition. Don't drink without eating. Carry salty snacks and munch regularly. You may also want to consider using a dilute electrolyte drink to help maintain the salts and electrolytes in your system as you exercise.

Chapter Seven

Illnesses

Illness in the field can be uncomfortable and scary. Most of us aren't doctors and can't tell the difference between a little bit of gas pain and a serious abdominal problem. Non-specific gastrointestinal distress—or a bellyache—is relatively common on camping trips, often as a result of poor hygiene. You can feel pretty lousy as a result of this, but it's not going to kill you. Appendicitis, on the other hand, might. Upper respiratory illnesses can be equally mysterious: Do you have a common cold or pneumonia? How can you tell when someone is seriously ill or simply uncomfortable?

Here are a few guidelines for helping you determine whether your patient needs to see a doctor. Try to make your patient comfortable and monitor him for twenty-four hours. If in doubt, get the person out. No one is going to criticize you for making a conservative call.

GUIDELINES FOR ASSESSING ILLNESSES

These guidelines will help you assess a person's illness:

Fever: Any illness associated with a fever for more than forty-eight hours should be considered

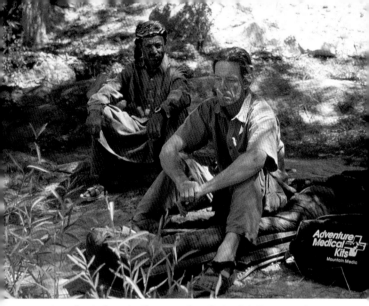

A moderate fever lasting more than forty-eight hours can be indicative of serious illness.

serious. High fevers are temperatures above 104°F and are often accompanied by delirium and convulsions, so you'll know it's bad. Moderate fevers between 102°F and 103°F for more than forty-eight hours are bad enough to consider evacuating your patient.

Breathing: For upper respiratory illnesses, any difficulty breathing that worsens over twenty-four hours may be a sign of more serious problems. Wheezing, shortness of breath, and anxiety are all potential signs of problems that demand medical attention. Monitor your patient and look for deterioration over time to help make your call.

Headache: Severe headaches that don't respond to pain medication, or persist over time and are accompanied by a stiff neck, are all potentially dangerous symptoms that should be evaluated by a medical professional.

Abdominal pain: Pain that worsens over twelve to twenty-four hours and/or is accompanied by a spiking fever, tensed muscles, tenderness or hardness in the belly on exam, and vomiting or diarrhea are signs that your patient may be suffering something more serious than simple gastrointestinal distress.

Vomiting/diarrhea: Inability to tolerate fluids or food for more than forty-eight hours.

If your patient exhibits one or more of these symptoms, seek medical help. If you are unsure, seek medical help.

Chapter Eight
Altitude Illness

As we all know, there's less oxygen at high elevations, so our bodies have to work harder to supply ourselves with enough air. We begin to feel the effects of elevation at around 8,000 feet, although real altitude illness is more common above 10,000 feet. Altitude illness baffles scientists. They know what happens, but they don't really know why some people suffer more than others. There's no real rhyme or reason: Young, strong athletes can get sick as easily as older, out-of-shape couch potatoes; and some people who have traveled to altitude in the past without problems fall ill on their next visit.

Your best bet for minimizing your risk is to ascend slowly and give your body time to adjust, or acclimate. Physicians recommend ascending at a rate of no more than 2,000 feet per day, with 1,500 feet being a more conservative measure.

Altitude illness is categorized as acute mountain sickness (AMS), high altitude cerebral edema (HACE), or high altitude pulmonary edema (HAPE). HACE and HAPE can be deadly. Often, but not always, your body will be showing some signs of AMS before you come down with HACE or HAPE, so it's important to recognize all the symptoms to protect yourself and your team from the problem.

AMS

Many people assume headaches are normal at altitude; they are not. A headache is one of the first and most classic signs that your body is feeling the effects of altitude and is having trouble adjusting. Other signs of AMS include nausea, lightheadedness, disturbed sleep, lethargy, and loss of coordination.

If you exhibit these signs, the best treatment is to stop ascending and give your body time to adapt to the elevation. Keep hydrated, try to eat, and do some light exercise. Once your body adjusts and your symptoms dissipate, you can continue to ascend.

HACE

HACE is swelling of the brain and can kill you quickly if not treated. Signs of HACE are changes in levels of consciousness, headache, nausea, vomiting, loss of muscle coordination, seizures, hallucinations, and vision disturbances.

Treatment is immediate descent. Symptoms will begin to abate as you lose elevation, but expect to go down 2,000 feet or more—until all signs are gone—to ensure your patient is safe.

HAPE

HAPE manifests itself in the lungs and is associated with shortness of breath even at rest, fatigue, dry cough progressing to a wet, productive cough, rattley breath sounds, and loss of muscle coordination.

As with HACE, the treatment for HAPE is to descend immediately and as quickly as possible. Again, symptoms will lessen as you go down.

With both HAPE and HACE, you can attempt to reascend once your patient is free of all symptoms of altitude illness. But go slowly and watch for signs of a reoccurrence. It's not worth risking your life for one more summit.

Drugs

There are medications available that help our bodies acclimate or alleviate symptoms of altitude illness, although most doctors recommend that you allow your body to adjust naturally. If, however, you are planning a trip to high elevations, you may want to consult a physician about the wisdom of carrying these drugs just in case you or someone in your group falls ill.

Chapter Nine

First-Aid Kit

Everyone has an opinion on what needs to be in a first-aid kit. The truth is, you never know. Your best bet is to think about items that are hard to duplicate: gel pads, athletic tape, medications. Leave behind things that can be improvised: cravats can be made from bandannas or T-shirts, bandages from gauze pads and tape.

On longer trips, a well-stocked first-aid kit allows you to deal with all sorts of illnesses and injuries.

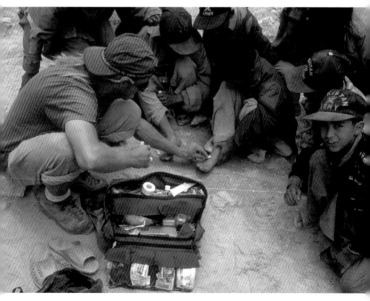

Factors that affect the size and extent of your kit include remoteness, length of stay, number of people, type of activity, and the presence of children. Try to keep things to a minimum. Big, bulky first-aid kits tend to be left in camp, where they do you absolutely no good.

Some useful items include the following:

- » Sterile gauze pads (assorted sizes)
- » ACE bandage
- » Occlusive dressing (e.g., Tegaderm)
- » Gel blister pads (assorted sizes)
- » Steri strips
- » 35-cc needle-nose syringe
- » 1.5-inch roll of athletic tape
- » Moleskin (one 4 x 7 sheet)
- » Second Skin
- » Trauma shears
- » Povidone-iodine
- » Topical antibiotic cream
- » Nonprescription pain medication (ibuprofen, acetaminophen, etc.)
- » Nonprescription antihistamine (Benedryl)
- » Gloves
- » Microshield or pocket mask
- » Notepad, pencil, emergency contact information

Optional items:

- » Gauze roll
- » Cortisone cream
- » Cravat or triangle bandage
- » Thermometer
- » Tweezers
- » Adhesive bandages
- » Soap-impregnated sponges
- » Epinephrine*
- » Antibiotics*
- » Diarrhea medication*

   *Consult with a doctor before using these medications.

Chapter Ten

A Final Word

Emergency situations are scary, especially if the person in trouble is your partner or child. Having a routine or prescribed set of steps to follow can help you stay calm and bring order to your situation. Here's where basic first aid helps. Not only does first aid give you the skills you need to help an injured or ill person, but it also provides guidance and structure to help control chaos and panic both in yourself and in those around you. Keep calm. Follow the basic steps outlined in this book and do the best you can.

When you are far from medical help, having some basic first-aid skills is imperative for coping with emergencies.

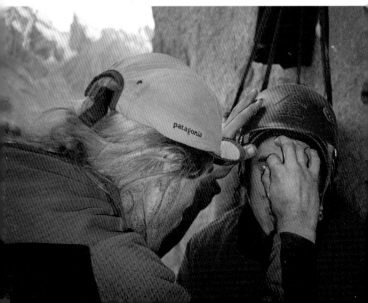

Index